LITTLE BOOK OF
MASSAGE

LITTLE BOOK OF
MASSAGE

First published in the UK in 2013

© Demand Media Limited 2013

www.demand-media.co.uk

Printed and bound in Europe.

ISBN 978-1-782811-85-5

The views in this book are those of the author but they are general views only and readers are urged to consult the relevant and qualified specialist for individual advice in particular situations.

Demand Media Limited hereby exclude all liability to the extent permitted by law of any errors or omissions in this book and for any loss, damage or expense (whether direct or indirect) suffered by a third party relying on any information contained in this book.

All our best endeavours have been made to secure copyright clearance for every photograph used but in the event of any copyright owner being overlooked please address correspondence to Demand Media Limited, Waterside Chambers, Bridge Barn Lane, Woking, Surrey, GU21 6NL

In no way will Demand Media Limited or any persons associated with Demand Media be held responsible for any injuries or problems that may occur during the use of this book or the advise contained within. We recommend that you consult a doctor before embarking any exercise programme. This product is for informational purposes only and is not meant as medical advice. Performing exercise of all types can pose a risk, know your physical limits, we suggest you perform adequate warm up and cool downs before and after any exercise. If you experience any pain, discomfort, dizziness or become short of breath stop exercising immediately and consult your doctor

Contents

Introduction

Massage is a natural therapy that can help treat many ills of everyday life that we all face. It is a very effective way of promoting good health, boosting circulation, lymph drainage, to release toxins and to thoroughly relax the mind and the body.

The Little Book of Massage gives you an insight into the techniques of Swedish massage so that you can try doing it to yourself, or to your family and friends.

Swedish massage uses five styles of long, flowing strokes to massage. The five basic strokes are 'effleurage' (sliding or gliding), 'petrissage' (kneading), 'tapotement' (rhythmic tapping), 'friction' (cross fibre) and vibration/shaking.

Swedish massage has shown to be helpful in reducing pain, joint stiffness, and improving function in patients with osteoarthritis of the knee over a period of eight weeks. The development of Swedish massage is often inaccurately credited to Per Henrik Ling, Swedish physical therapist, developer and teacher of medical-gymnastics. It was in fact the Dutch practitioner Johan Georg Mezger who adopted the French names to denote the basic strokes. The term 'Swedish' massage is actually only recognised in English and Dutch speaking countries, and in Hungary. Elsewhere (including Sweden) the style is referred to as 'classic massage'.

This book features Victoria Sprigg CIBTAC, MISPA, IIHHT, a holistic therapist who uses Swedish massage to great effect in treating a variety of health problems. Her programme Swedish Massage – The Complete Body Experience is also available on DVD to complement this volume.

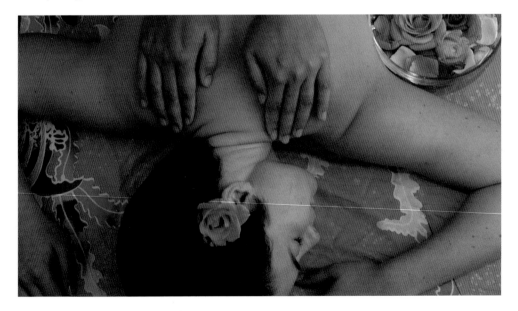

The Swedish Massage

The person being massaged should always be kept completely covered, except for the limb being massaged. Always use plenty of oil, otherwise the skin tends to stick to the hand and will cause too much friction.

When massaging any area you never remove your hands from the body; you should always be in contact with at least one hand. The only exception to this is when you have just finished a particular area, or are adjusting towels on the body.

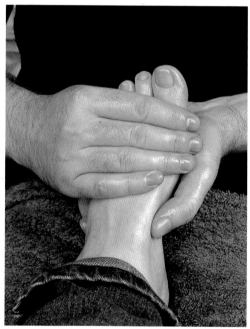

Those who should not have Swedish massage are perhaps the very elderly, the frail, those with very high blood pressure or anyone recuperating from recent operations, or pregnant ladies who would find it difficult lying on their stomachs.

Chapter 1

The Front of the Legs

Always start work on the front of the body, starting on one leg and using plenty of oil to massage upwards towards the heart. This sliding or gliding movement is called effleurage and consists of a firm stroke upwards and then coming lightly back down followed by a little tug. Massage the leg for a minute or so.

Step 1   Step 2

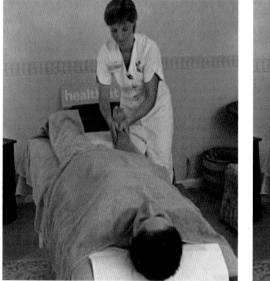

Push any toxins down the quadriceps, upwards towards the lymph node in the groin area.

Step 1   Step 2

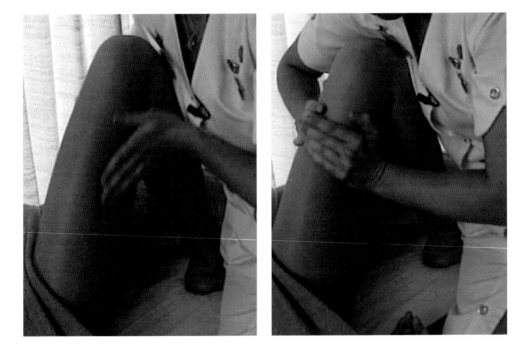

Using your knuckles pushing any toxins upwards along the hamstrings at the back of the thigh.

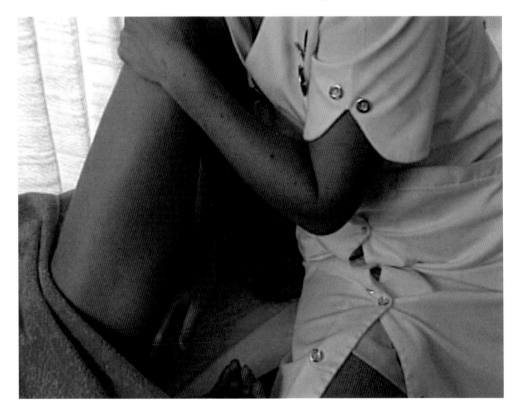

Give the leg a tug to stretch it before laying it down and covering it up.

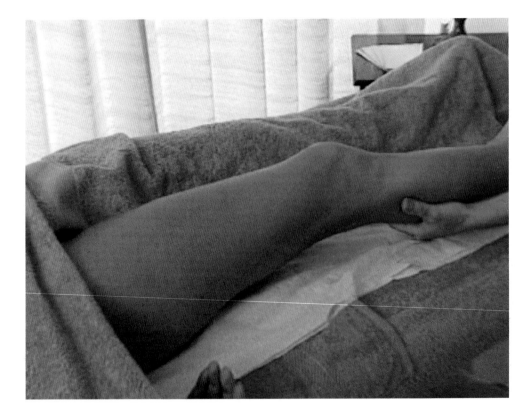

Massaging any of the joints is a wonderful feeling. It really warms the area as well as draining any toxins.

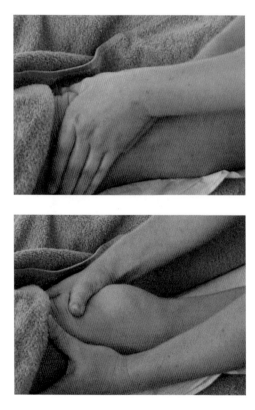

Step 1

Step 2

Also use your thumbs to push any toxins from this area and then down to the lymph node at the back of the knee.

Step 1

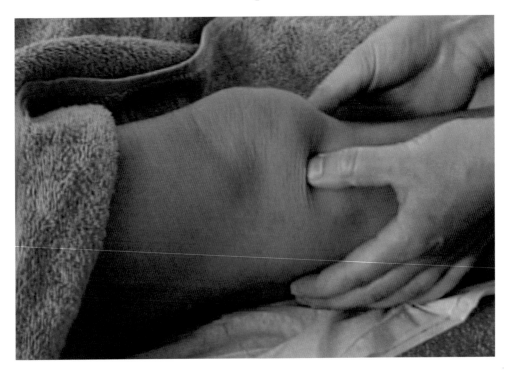

Step 2

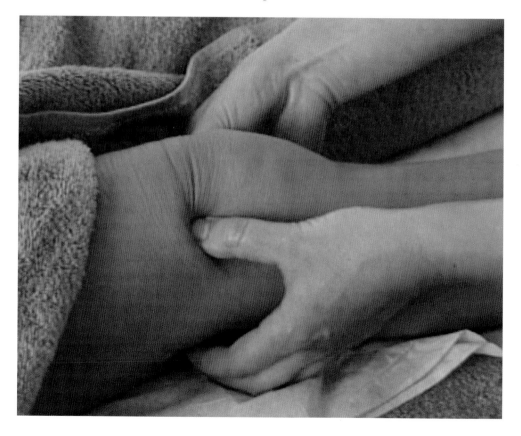

Step 3

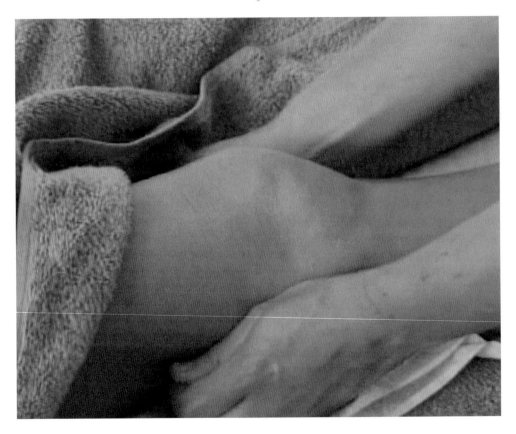

Moving onto the ankle, circle the joint in both directions to mobilise it nicely.

Step 1   Step 2

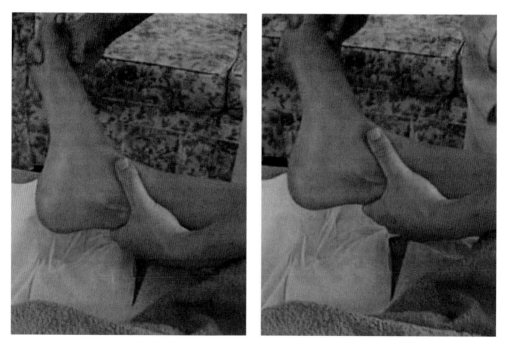

Smooth out all the toxins around the joint.

Step 1   Step 2

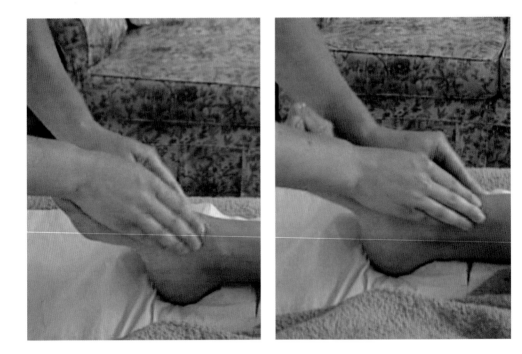

Then coming up the foot, doing the petrissage movement between the metatarsal bones which connect the toes, push all the toxins away.

Step 1   Step 2

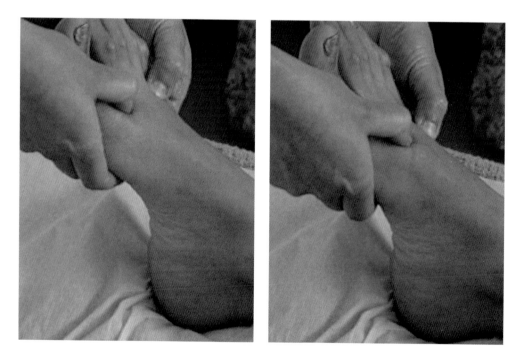

Massage behind the foot and then stretching the toes.

Step 1

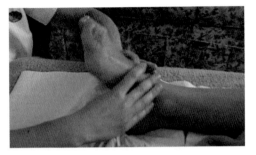

Step 2

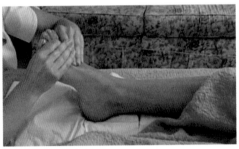

Step 3

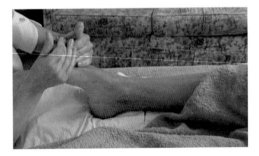

Massage underneath the foot again using the technique shown in the pictures. All the nerve endings and energy lines in line with reflexology will be massaged.

Step 1

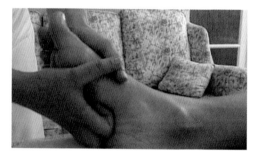

Step 2

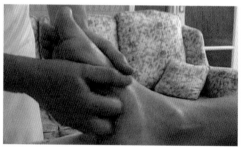

Step 3

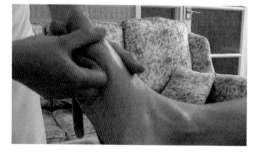

Repeat on the other leg.

When complete, cover both legs up to make them feel warm and secure. Also now place a pillow under the thighs and knees of the person, which makes them feel very secure and also releases any pressure from the lower back.

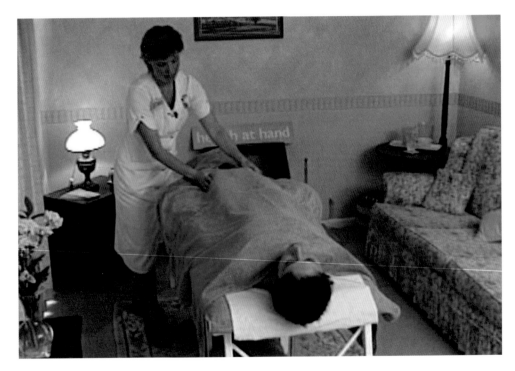

Chapter 2

Stomach

Only reveal the area to be massaged and them warm more oil in your hands.

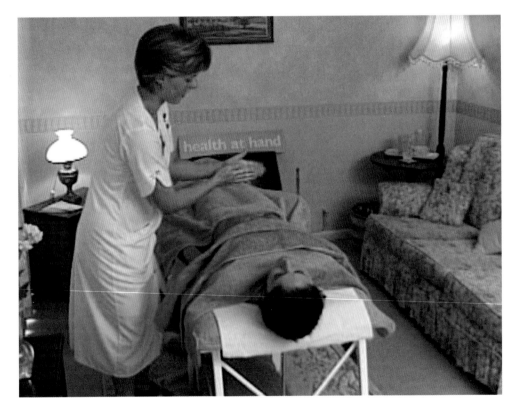

The stomach area demonstrates why a therapist needs to know anatomy and physiology in depth because of the digestive system. You massage in the direction of the colon from the lower right hand area round in an upside-down horseshoe shape to the lower left hand area.

Step 1

Step 2

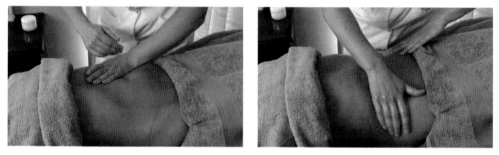

Step 3

Step 4

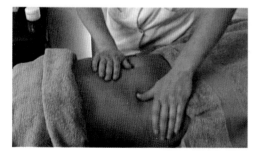
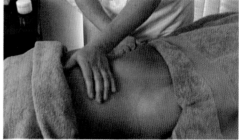

Massage down the sides making a nice pull-up towards the hips.

Step 1   Step 2

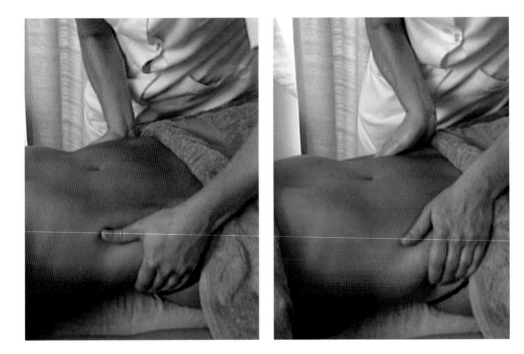

Finish the area with the effleurage movement around the stomach and then cover it up again.

Step 1   Step 2

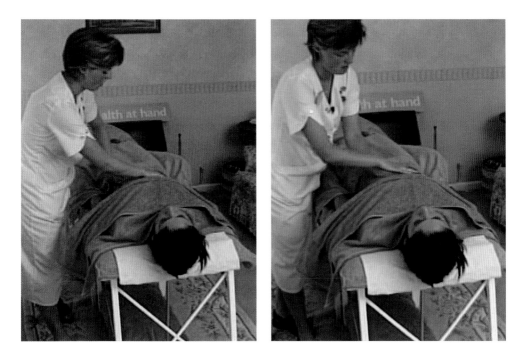

Chapter 3

The Arms

Just reveal the one arm, making sure that the rest of the body is nice and warm.

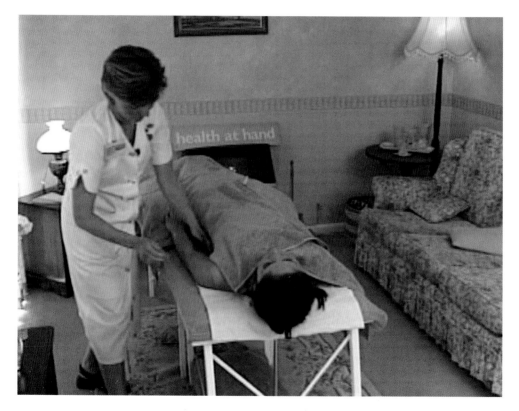

Introduce the oil to the body and massage the arm up and down using the same effleurage movement already used on the leg. Massage for ten seconds or so.

Step 1

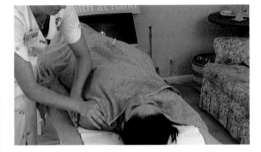

Step 2

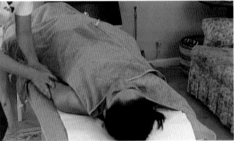

Step 3

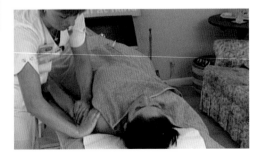

Bring the arm up and massage it in the same way in this position. This is a nice movement because gravity is helping you to push all the toxins down towards the lymph node under the armpit.

Step 1

Step 2

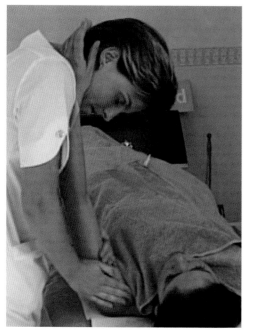 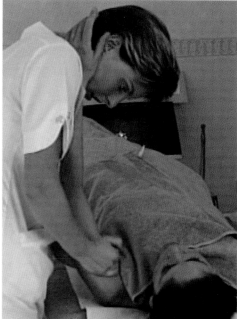

Put the arm down and give it a little tug.

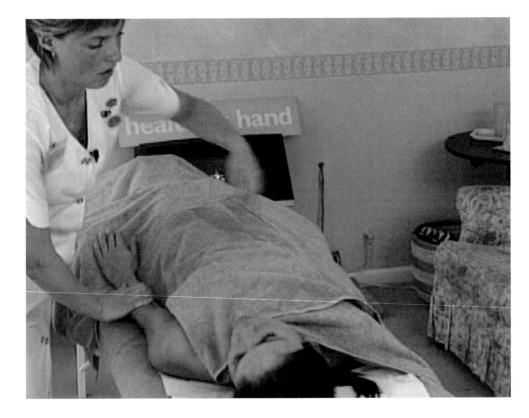

Working on the mobility of the shoulder joint, gently rotate the shoulder one way and then the other, holding onto the arm as shown.

Step 1   Step 2

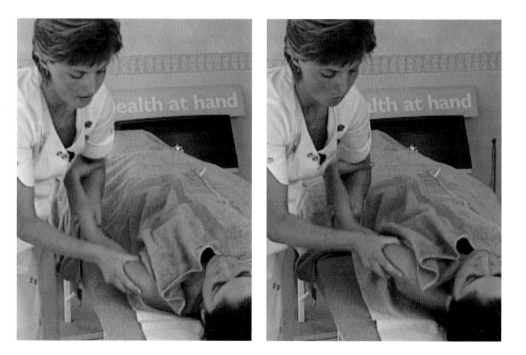

With the person totally relaxed and allowing their arm to completely flop, move it backwards and forwards, as shown, as a flexibility exercise.

Step 1   Step 2

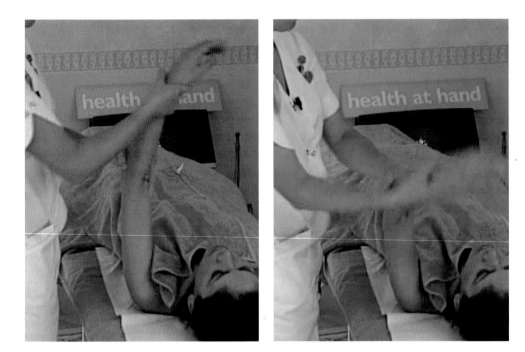

Finish with a gentle tug when the arm is back down by the side.

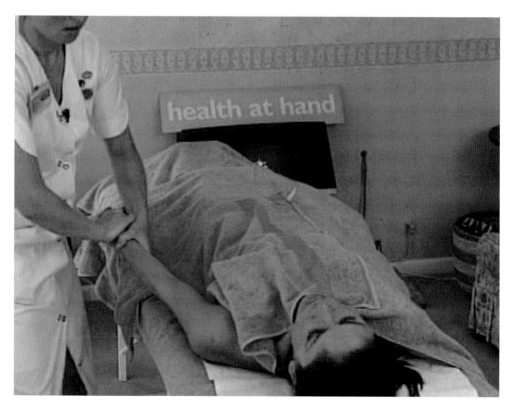

Working on the forearm, place the upper arm and elbow on the bed and hold the hand up. Massage the forearm moving from the wrist down towards the elbow.

Step 1   Step 2

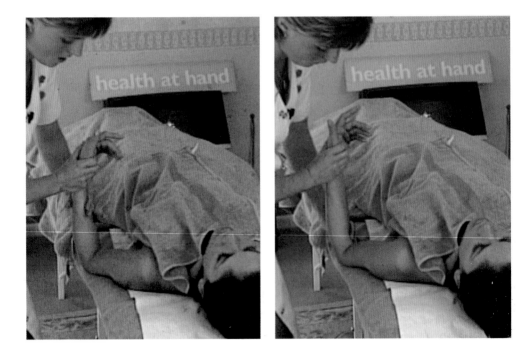

You can also squeeze the forearm moving down.

Step 1   Step 2

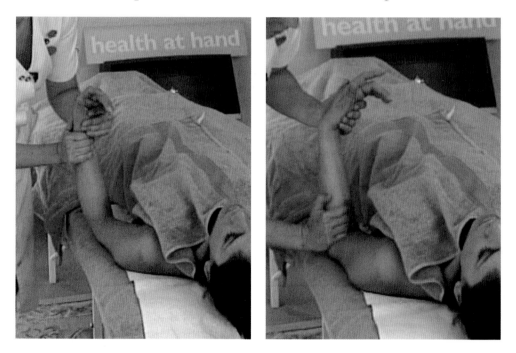

Finish with further effleurage for a few seconds.

Cover up the upper arm before starting work on the wrist and the hand. Rotate the wrist for a few seconds.

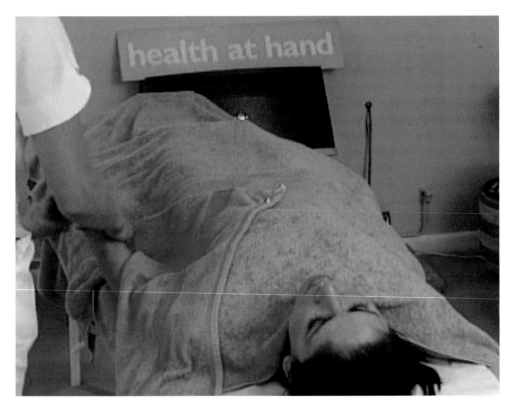

Massage the wrist always pushing the fluid to the back and then towards the elbow where the nearest lymph node is situated.

Step 1

Step 2

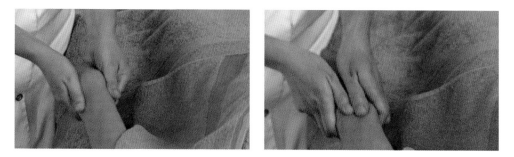

Step 3

Step 4

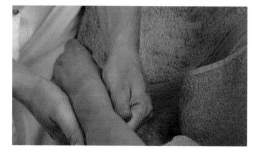
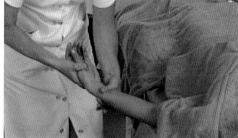

Work the hand just the same as the foot by pushing the fluid between
the metacarpals from the base of the fingers towards the wrist.

Step 1   Step 2

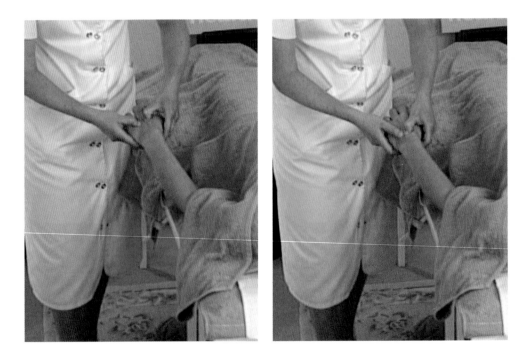

Massage each finger followed by a rotation and then a gentle tug.

Step 1

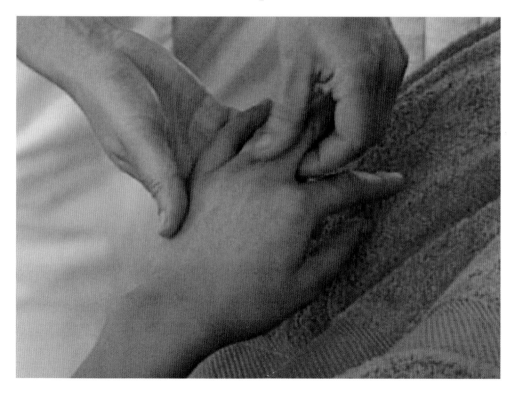

Step 2

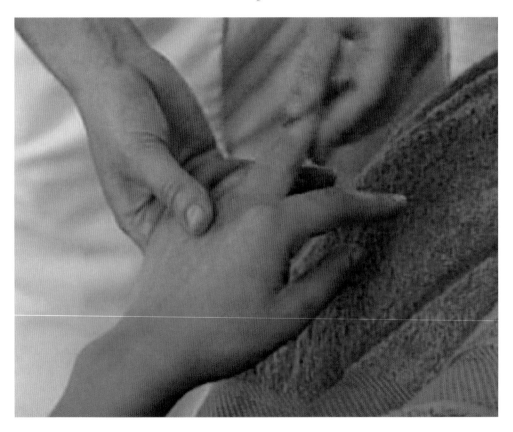

Step 3

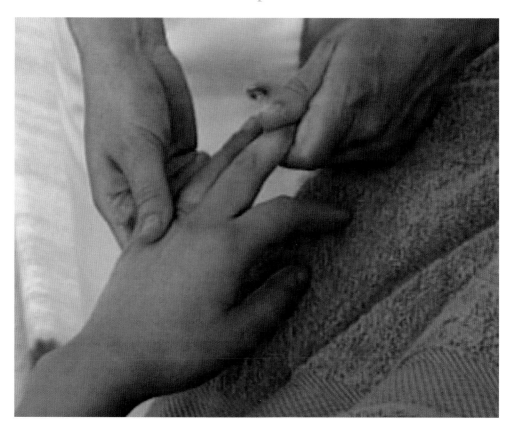

Turn the palm over and stretch the hand out.

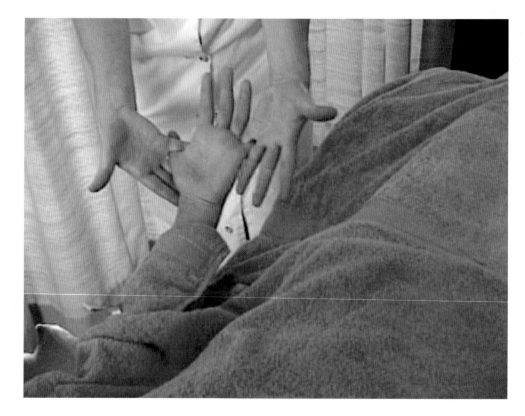

Using your thumbs to massage alternately the centre of the palm.

Step 1   Step 2

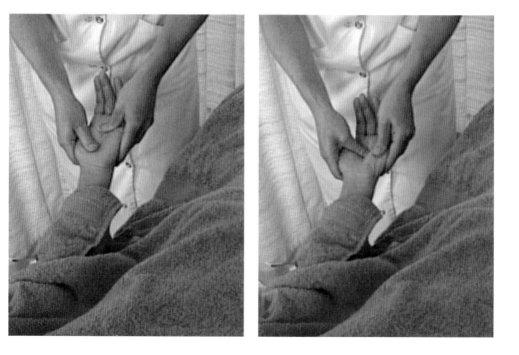

This area in reflexology terms is called the solar plexus, which on our bodies is located as shown and is the centre of our emotions and feelings.

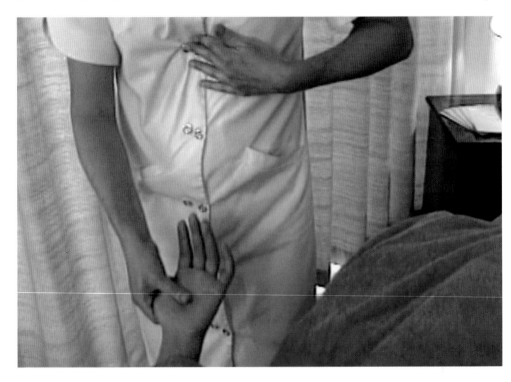

Cover the hand and repeat with the other arm.

Ask the person to turn over onto their front, holding the towel as shown and remove the pillow from under the legs.

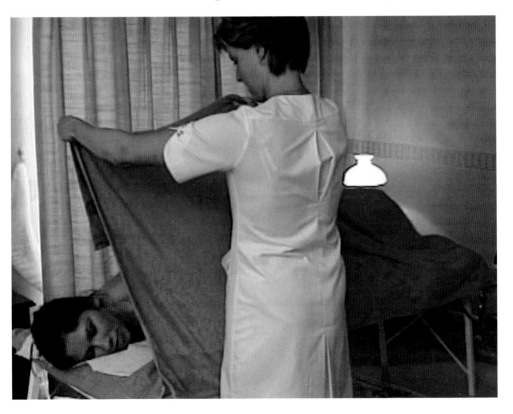

Chapter 4

Back of the Legs

Uncover the limb to be worked on. Massage the back of the leg with the effleurage movement for a minute or so.

Step 1

Step 2

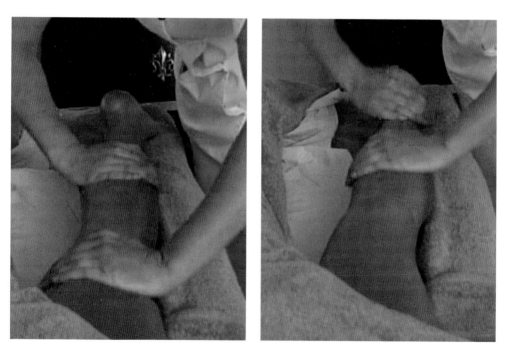

Work on the lower leg with your thumbs, first on the Achilles tendon, then working up the back of the calf muscle. Push upwards towards the knee, which pushes all the toxins towards the lymph node behind the knee.

Step 1

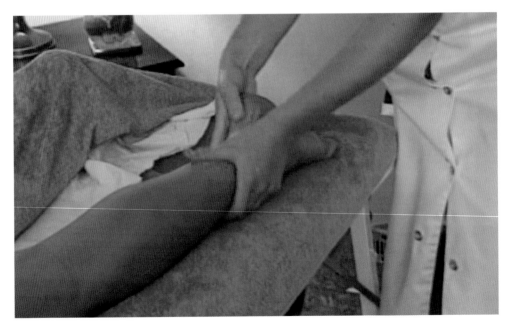

Step 2

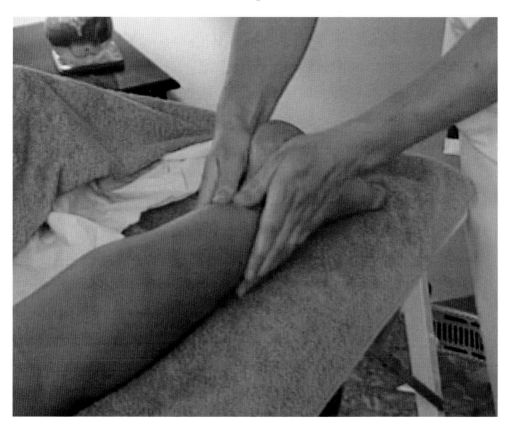

Step 3

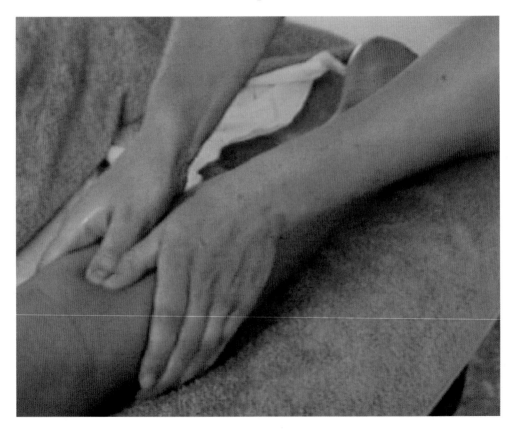

Work the inner thigh by first of all making sweeping movements with your hands upwards.

Step 1   Step 2

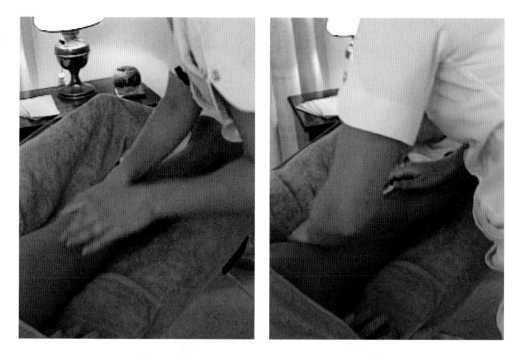

Then knead the area.

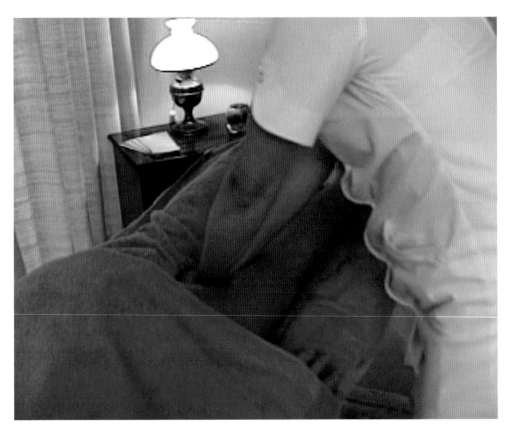

This is followed by some squeezing by picking up the muscle.

Step 1   Step 2

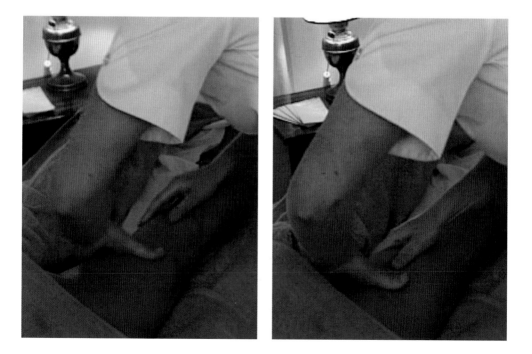

Move round to the other side of the bed so that the upper thigh can be worked on. Start by doing some squeezing movements as before.

Step 1   Step 2

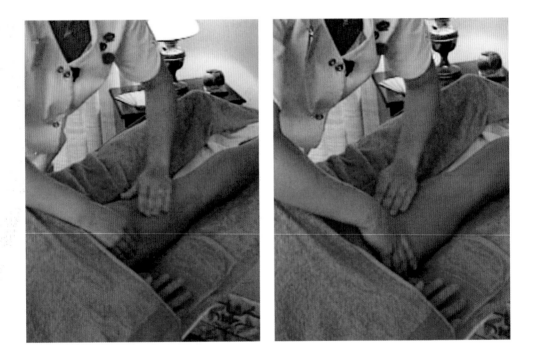

Follow this by kneading the area.

Step 1

Step 2

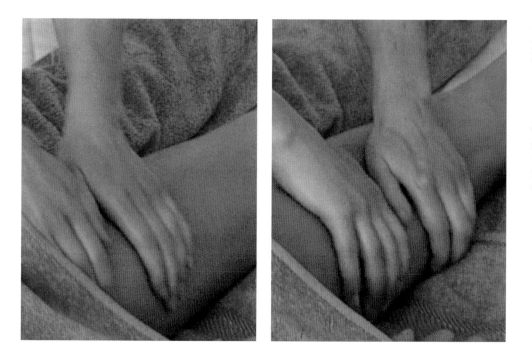

Another technique is now introduced – the percussion movement – which is achieved by using the hand, in a cup shape, and fingertips to tap quickly and quite firmly on the area being treated – called 'cupping'. This progresses to using the side of the hand in the same rapid movements – called 'hacking'. The percussion movement is excellent for cellulite.

Step 1   Step 2

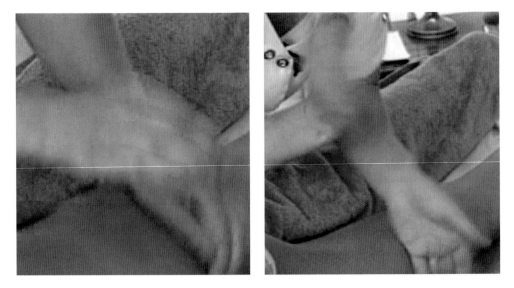

Massage up the side of the hip and up to the buttock using your thenar
muscle strongly to bring the circulation upwards and into the centre of
the buttock.

Step 1   Step 2

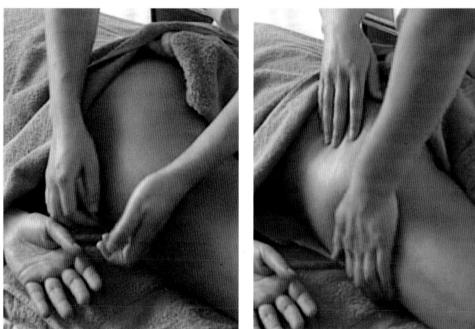

Move to using a technique called petrissage (see image shown). Massage firmly into the centre of the buttock

Step 1   Step 2

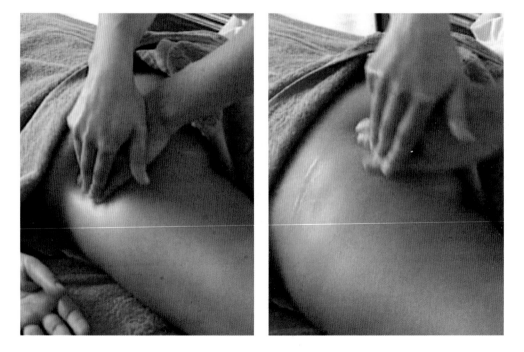

Finish this area by using the squeezing movement and then kneading and then back to the percussion moves, first cupping and then hacking as already shown.

Step 1 Step 2

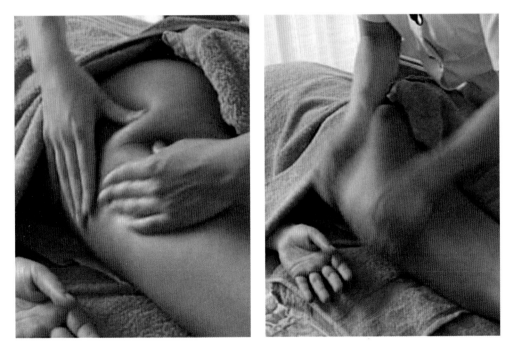

Finish the back of that leg by doing some nice long effleurage movements to tell the whole leg that you are still there. Then raise the lower leg and perform some sweeps down the back of the calf muscle.

Step 1 Step 2

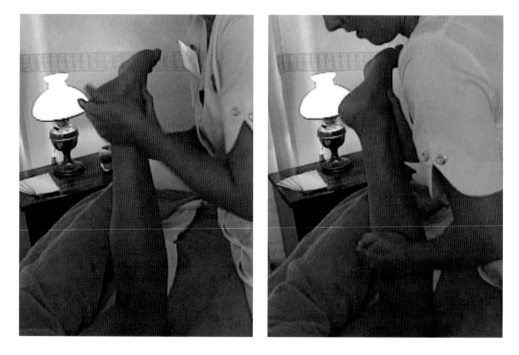

Apply some pressure to the sole of the foot before placing the leg back down.

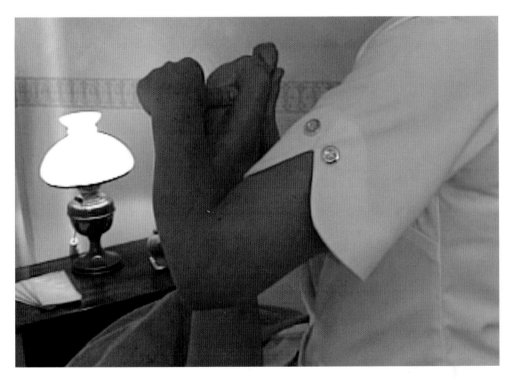

Cover this leg and repeat on the other one.

Chapter 5

The Back and Shoulders

Uncover the back area, tucking the towel in and applying some oil.

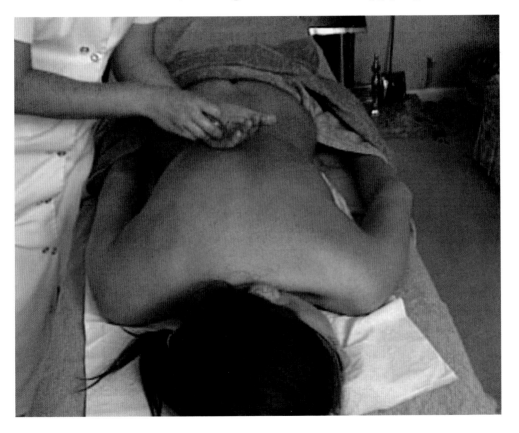

Ask the person to take a deep breath in and as they exhale stretch the spine lengthways with each hand going in opposite directions. This stretches all of the vertebra out in a movement that can't be done by yourself.

Step 1   Step 2

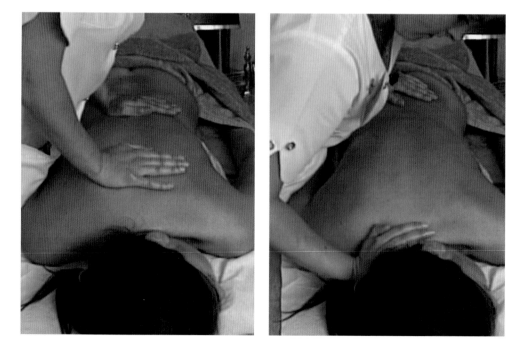

Stretch all the way up the back using effleurage with both hands starting at the base of the spine, moving up to the shoulders. Use your palms only; don't press your fingers in.

Step 1

Step 2

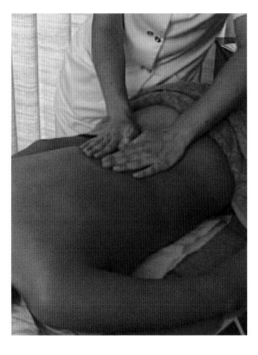

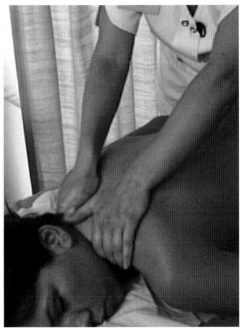

Coming up to the shoulder, take the arm and place and hold it behind the back. Massage the shoulder blade and then perform some deep petrissage movements on the area.

Step 1

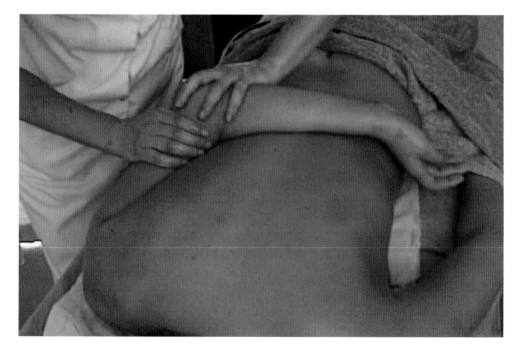

Step 2

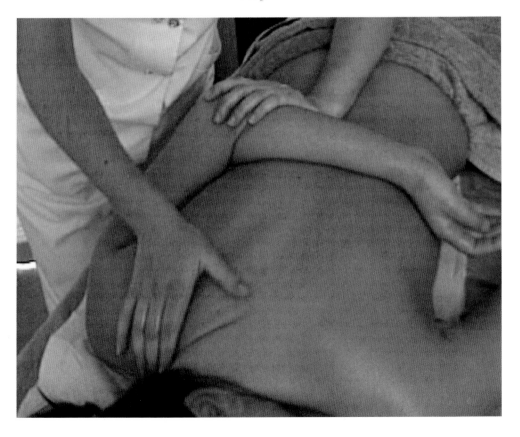

Step 3

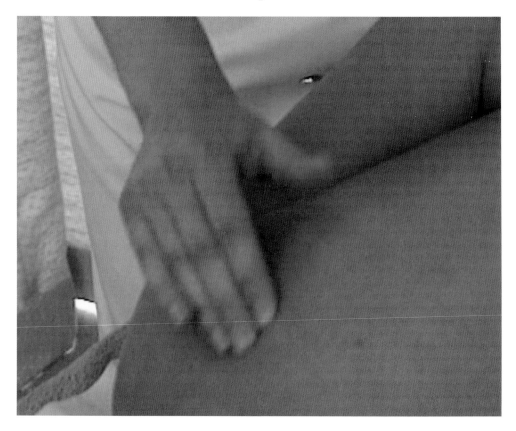

LITTLE BOOK OF **MASSAGE**

Release all the pressure by doing a palm movement over the shoulder before releasing the arm back down again.

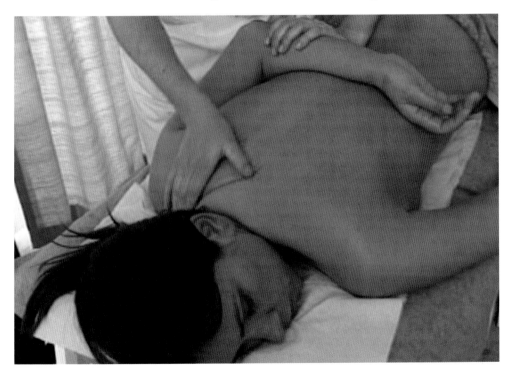

Repeat on the other shoulder.

Introduce your hands back to the body and stretch all the way up the back using effleurage with both hands starting at the base of the spine, moving up to the shoulders.

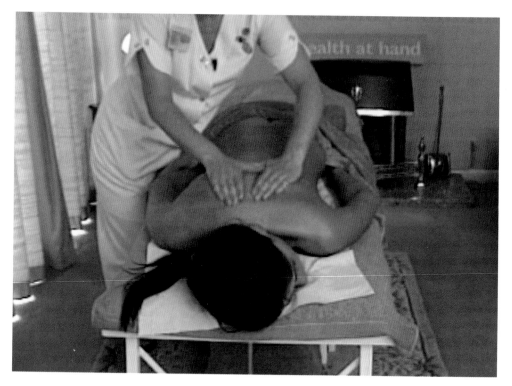

Perform percussion moves round the circle of the body; start by squeezing first of all as seen earlier on the legs.

Step 1   Step 2

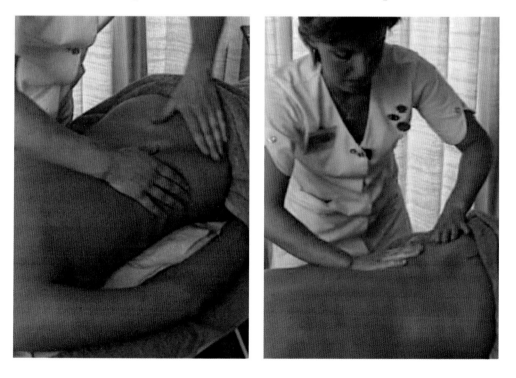

Move to kneading round the whole area before moving onto the percussion moves – cupping first and then hacking. Go round the body circle twice for each movement.

Step 1

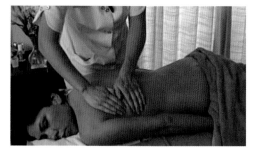

Step 2

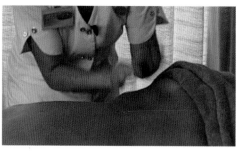

Step 3

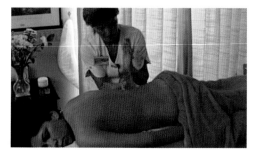

Return to effleurage with both hands starting at the base of the spine to calm the body again after the quite physical movements just performed.

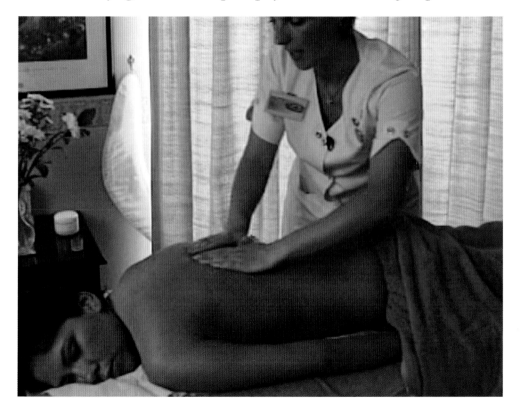

Coming to the base of the spine, this area is like a plate and quite often harbours toxins. Massage the area using your thumbs.

Step 1   Step 2

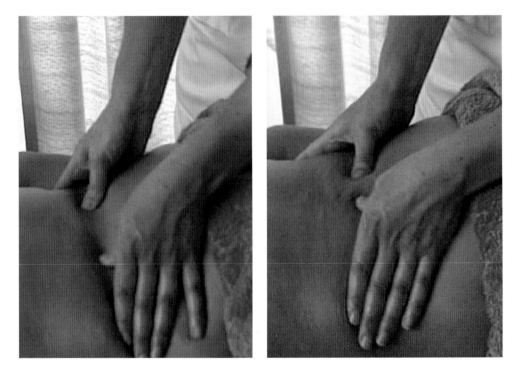

Then work upwards all the way to the top of the neck, again using your thumbs.

Step 1   Step 2

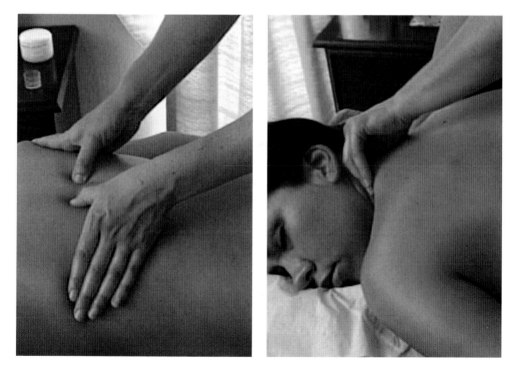

This is repeated by using a different movement called 'vibration'. With the hand position shown, move up the spine a little at a time and every time you stop make a small but vigorous sideways movement with your hand to 'vibrate' each area.

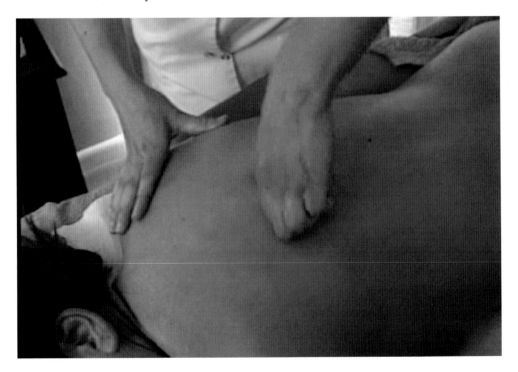

Finish off with a hip stretch, a thoracic stretch and a shoulder stretch.

Step 1

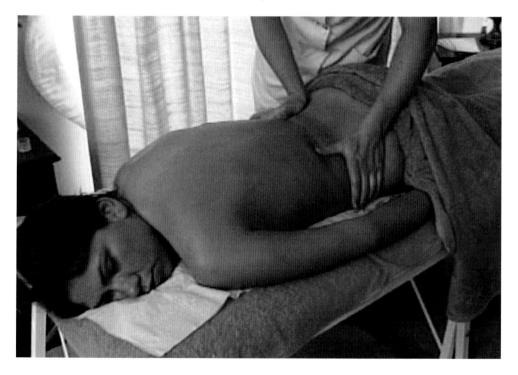

Step 2

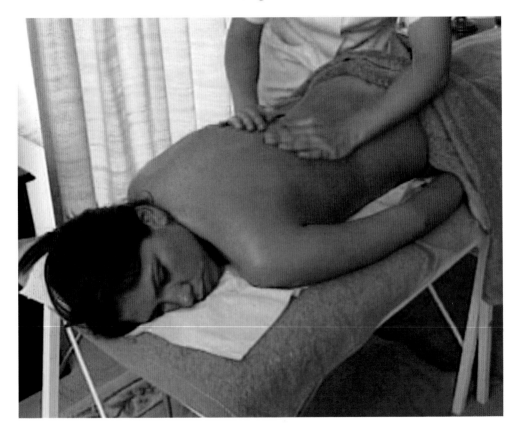

Step 3

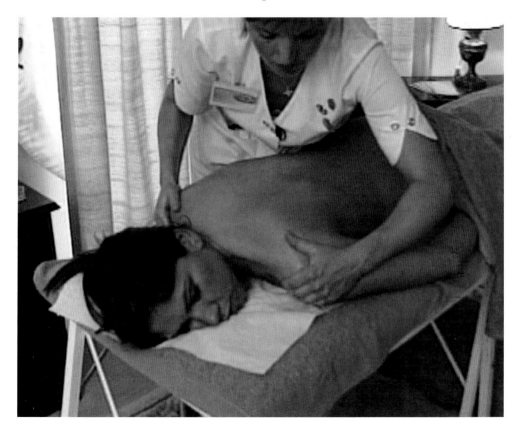

Always complete with effleurage and one final back spine stretch.

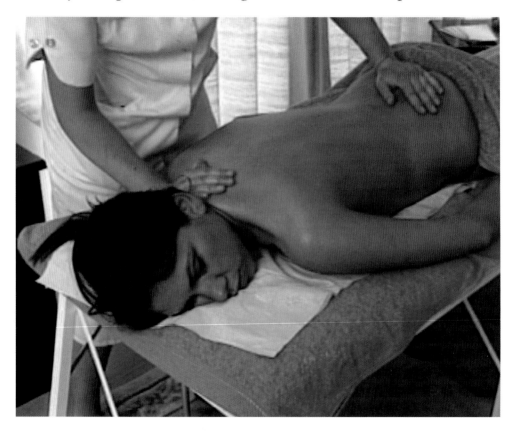

Chapter 6

Chest, Shoulders and Neck

Ask the person to turn over again onto their back. Place the pillow back under the knees and wrap their legs and feet up properly.

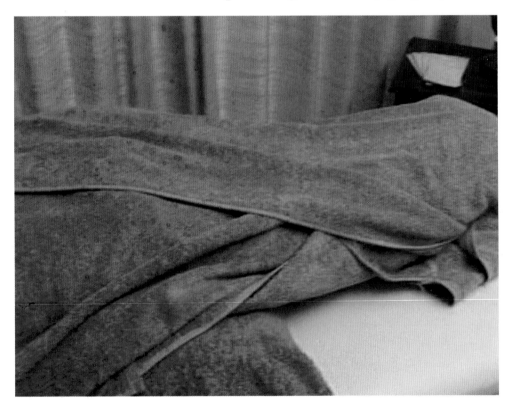

Introduce the hands to the chest area, putting oil all over. Use a flowing effleurage movement working down over the clavicle, down the sternum, over the shoulder points and then a nice firm movement underneath and pulling the neck.

Step 1

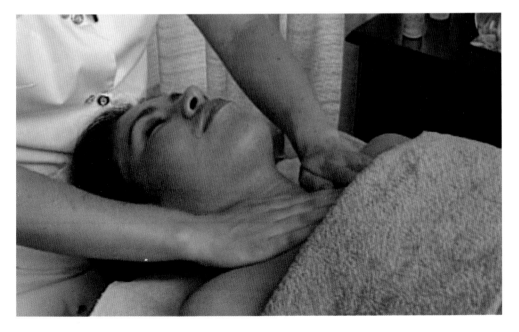

Step 2

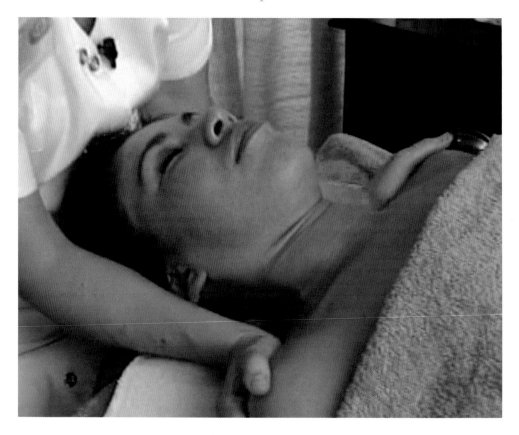

Step 3

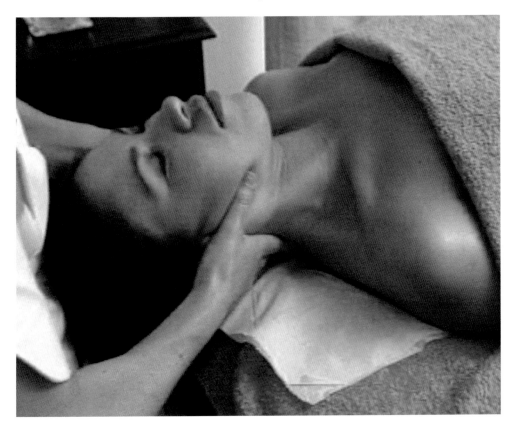

Massage with your knuckles over the chest and round the shoulders. This area collects a lot of tension, so it needs a good firm massage.

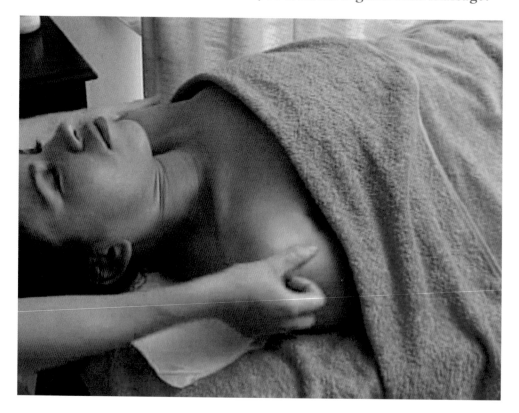

Working again first on the chest area use a movement called 'tapotement', which is a rhythmic tapping technique using the tips of the fingers. Even though this is a really light massage, it decongests the upper chest area all the way to the lungs of any toxins; very good for any chest problems, bronchitis, asthma, even sore throats and congested chests.

Step 1   Step 2

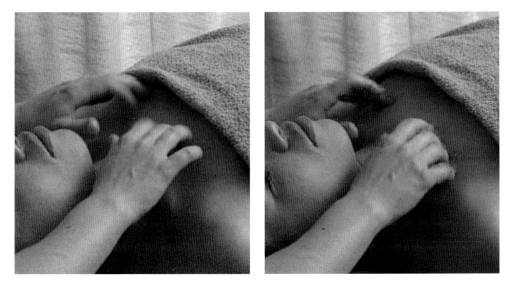

Turn the head to the side and ask the person to relax completely; the more they relax the more benefit they will get out of it. Stretch round the shoulder and back up, just gently pulling the head up. Your other hand should be under the other side of the head so that it is completely supported.

Step 1   Step 2

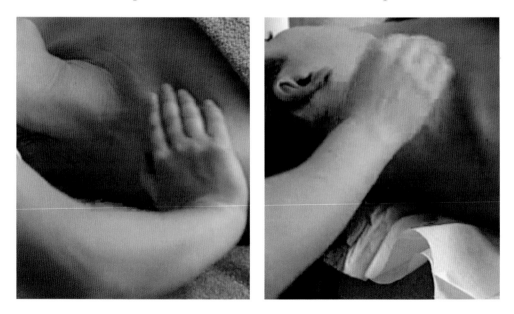

Gently start knuckling the shoulder area, use the whole of the hand with all fingers knuckling together.

Step 1   Step 2

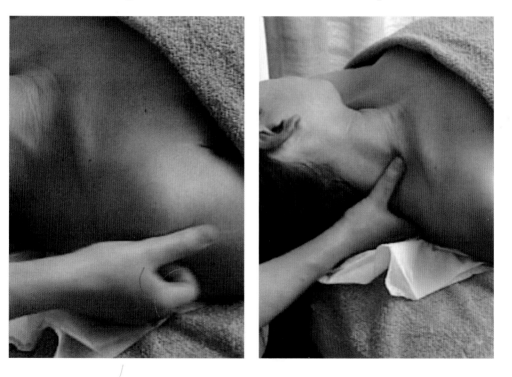

Finish with a stretch of the neck and effleurage out from the shoulder back up to the neck to bring all the toxins that have just been massaged out, up. Then bring the head back to centre.

Step 1   Step 2

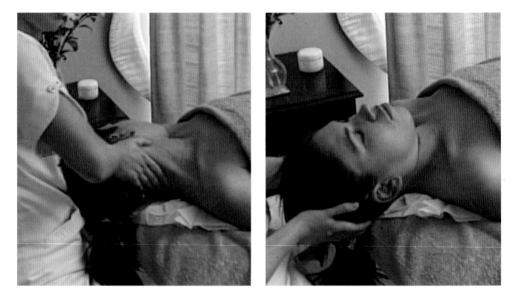

Turn the person's head to the other side and repeat the above, now incorporating the opposite shoulder.

Moving to focus on the neck, start by performing a nice neck stretch. Lift the head and use two fingers of each hand to massage upwards from the spine, bringing up all the toxins. Rest the head gently back down.

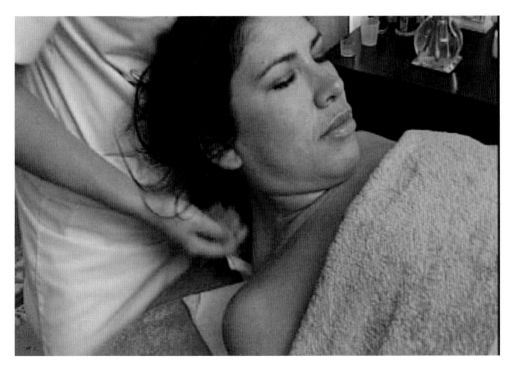

Finish the whole session by coming up round the scalp and off.

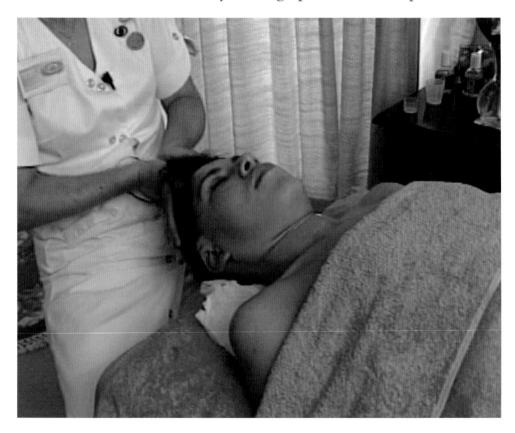

Cover the exposed upper body with the towel and to complete the session properly, hold the shoulders down, which releases any pressure. Because the person is covered up it tells them that that is the end of the massage.

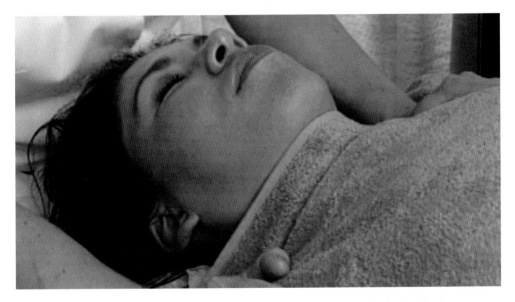

This is a typical Swedish massage that covers the whole body but stops at the neck, whereas with other massages the face, the scalp and the back of the head can be incorporated.

Design and artwork by Scott Giarnese

Published by Demand Media Limited

Publishers Jason Fenwick & Jules Gammond

Written by Michelle Brachet